Heart

Michael Carl Brabeck

This story is dedicated to my wife, Mary, who has urged me for more than thirty years to write it, and has given me the confidence to finally do it.

Preface

I am the second of four boys in a family normal in every way but for Steve. Stephen Joseph Brabeck's congenital heart disease—his and his family's experience of it—dominated the landscape of my childhood and was the central theme of our family life as we boys were growing up. Our parents' refusal to accept the inevitability of Steve's early death, and their tenacity in seeking to save him, enabled his survival. This is a story of his cure and the restoration of his future. It is tale that of necessity recounts the tireless efforts of many investigators and the brilliance and courage of a few surgeons, through whose efforts definitive cure of these defects finally became possible.

I originally conceived of writing this story to memorialize my mother and father, Marie and George, two truly wonderful human beings. Our present family and all who come after should know who these two people were.

My sources for the narrative are newspaper accounts, original articles and essays in medical journals spanning the years 1955-2005, and, most important, interviews with my brothers Tom, Pete, and Steve.

I will be ever grateful for having been born into this family.

MCB
December 5, 2009

Family

It's a crisp late-March morning as I drive south on US 52. This is southeastern Minnesota farm country, the heartland. The fields are dark and barren, the stubble of last year's growth broken occasionally by a naked tree, a rock-strewn ridge, or a lonely disc harrow, which seems to be awaiting the arrival of spring. On the four-lane I speed by the towns of Cannon Falls, Zumbrota, and Pine Island. I imagine the highway as it was when it consisted of only two lanes and passed directly through these small farming towns.

The sun slowly climbs in the southeast, causing a hard, flat glare through the windshield that makes me wish I had not forgotten to bring my sunglasses from home.

Home is New York City, where I live and work. I am a general internist, a hospitalist in the Department of Medicine at Bellevue Hospital Center, an old and storied public hospital on Manhattan's East Side. To see me as a patient, you must be in a horizontal position, admitted to an inpatient bed.

Once, my mother and father made this drive to bring their five-year-old child, Stevie, to Rochester. Their destination was the famed Mayo Clinic. The sum of their hopes was bundled with their little boy in the car that morning. Nearly fifty-two years later, it is I who am driving from St. Paul to Rochester. I am going to meet Steve and his wife, Lisi, at the Clinic. Steve has come for his second heart surgery there, which is scheduled the next day. Steve has known for most of his adult life that he would eventually have to return.

Turning down the radio's volume, I begin to think about 1955 and about my mother. Winston Churchill resigned in April of that year, Juan Peron was ousted in a military *coup d'état* in Argentina, and Dwight Eisenhower, in the third year of his two-term presidency, suffered a heart attack and was hospitalized for three weeks. Martin Lu-

1

ther King led a bus boycott in Montgomery, Alabama, the first major event of the U.S. civil rights movement. Disneyland opened in Anaheim, California, and the labor unions AFL and CIO merged. The biggest sports story of the year was the defeat of the New York Yankees by the Brooklyn Dodgers in the seventh and deciding game of the World Series.

But on September 12, the redemption of Brooklyn had yet to occur. It was eight o'clock in the evening, twilight time for that season. I imagine that in St. Paul the autumn evenings were still mild. I can see Mom seated in the enclosed back porch of our house on Highland Parkway. She is watching television while ironing our next day's school uniforms. The phone rings. It is her oldest and closest friend, Peg Maykoski. "Marie," Peg says, "Turn the TV to Channel 2. A Mayo Clinic doctor is talking about heart surgery there. They're talking about exactly the type of problems that Stevie has." My mother reaches to turn the dial on the set. She switches to *Medical Horizons*, the first nationally broadcast program ever to originate from Rochester, Minnesota. She listens with focused attention as the interviewer questions a bespectacled, rather bookish-looking young surgeon, John W. Kirklin, about a series of eight children with congenital heart disease on whom he and his colleagues at the Mayo Clinic have operated. The goal was definitive correction of their cardiac defects. Four of the eight patients have died. The others left the hospital cured.

Two weeks later, my mother and father, with Stevie, drove the ninety miles from St. Paul to Rochester, not yet knowing that this trip was the first leg of a journey that would give him back his future.

When they married, my parents wanted to start a family right away, as Mom was already twenty-eight years old. A former high school teacher and at that time a stay-at-home housewife, she wanted a daughter, as did my father. He was away from home a lot while we were growing up, on the road selling gloves and knitted caps to jobbers in every state west of the Mississippi. He described himself as a manufacturer's representative. We boys called him a traveling salesman. We said he lived out of the trunk of his car.

Their wish for a girl notwithstanding, Mom and Dad eventually got four boys instead: Pete, Mike, Tom, and Stevie.

Pete arrived in 1942, three years after their marriage and about a year after Mom received a medical opinion that she would never be able to conceive. My parents asked Mom's friend, Peg, to be his godmother. Their joy at his birth was undiminished by Pete's harelip and cleft palate, which required him to have bottle feedings until the lip and palate defects were surgically corrected. As a toddler Pete began speech therapy supervised by Sister Anna Marie at her school on Summit Avenue in St. Paul. A nun in the St. Paul Province of the order of the Sisters of St. Joseph of Carondelet, she was an early innovator in therapy for children with speech impediments,

Mom loved classical music, and our RCA Victor phonograph in the living room was in constant use. Pete was a bright child, and by the age of two he was able to identify Beethoven's Choral and Pastoral symphonies as well as several Mozart concertos.

Pete was the only focus of Mom's life in his first two years. That changed when I arrived in 1944, then Tom in 1947. Tom was different from the start. A photograph of him when he was about nine months old, suspended in a baby jumping chair with his toes just touching the floor, shows a wild-eyed, wire-haired blondie, his small fists gripping the metal frame of the tray at his chest, looking as if he were going to launch himself from that contraption at any second. From his youngest days Tom was a spark of energy and ebullience in our family, always first in fun, jokes, and laughter, and frequently first in trouble. One time, during a spanking ("Down the basement with you! I'm going to teach you a lesson!"), Dad was surprised on the first whack, when, instead of compliant buttock flab, the palm of his hand struck Tom's flat, unforgiving backside in a loud *thwack*! Reaching inside Tom's trousers, he retrieved a recent issue of *Time* magazine.

Stephen Joseph Brabeck was born on April 9, 1950, the last of the four boys. Shortly after Stevie's birth, Mom and Dad brought him to our family pediatrician for a well baby check. Dr. Steinberg immediately noted a harsh, ominous-sounding heart murmur and referred him to a pediatric heart specialist at the University of Minnesota's Variety Club Heart Hospital. Variety Club, perched high on the east bank of the Mississippi River in Minneapolis, was the first hospital in the United States to specialize exclusively in heart disease. Its pediatric cardiologists cared for many children with congenital heart defects, for which there was no cure available at that time. The consultation there revealed a constellation of congenital heart defects called Tetralogy of Fallot. Because there was no effective treatment for this condition, survival beyond adolescence of a "Tet kid," as they were called, was rare.

Mom had faced only two crises in her life before Steve's illness. The first was the death of her younger sister, Ida, at age six. Ida developed an earache, and several days later died of meningitis, which in the pre-antibiotic era was the most dreaded complication of an ear infection. When Mom recounted this to us boys, it was but a distant memory for her. But her father, apparently, never fully recovered from the loss. She told us that for the rest of his life he would suddenly begin to sob at the mere thought of Ida, who died in his arms.

Mom's second crisis occurred when she was in her early twenties. Born to German immigrants in 1911, she obtained master of arts degrees in German literature from the University of Minnesota and in music from the College of St. Catherine in St. Paul. She was also an accomplished pianist. In 1934, when she was 23 years old, she placed first in a national piano competition. The award was a scholarship for one year of study in Vienna with the renowned Austrian classical pianist Artur Schnabel. However, her father, who was business manager for the St. Paul-based Catholic newspaper, *Der Wanderer*, was politically well informed. Anticipating that war would soon break out in Europe, he refused to allow her to claim the prize. Marie was devastated. Years later, when we boys were grown and had our own families, she still spoke occasionally of her disappointment, which seemed to have faded little with the years. Despite these early trials, I think Mom would have said she led a charmed life in her youth. That is, until Steve was born with congenital heart disease.

Blue Baby

Niels Stensen, a Dane, is credited with the first description of Tetralogy of Fallot in 1671. The syndrome, however, is named for Louis Arthur Fallot, the French physician who published an account of two patients with the condition in 1888 in a paper titled *"Contribution a l'anatomie pathologique de la maladie bleu (cyanose cardique)."*

The heart is fundamentally a complicated muscular pump. In simplest terms, it is a four-chambered structure, with two chambers (the atria) for receiving venous blood and two (the ventricles) for pumping blood forward into the arteries. The right atrium and ventricle are separated from their left-sided counterparts by a muscular partition called the septum. The right atrium passively receives oxygen-poor blood from the body's veins and then delivers it to the right ventricle, which pumps it to the lungs so that it can be freshly oxygenated. With its replenished supply of oxygen, the blood flows directly back into the heart's left atrium, and from there it passes to the left ventricle. Through a squeezing action called systole, the richly oxygenated blood is expelled from the left ventricle and delivered to the arteries. Imagine for a moment a tree: the aorta is the trunk of the tree, which branches successively into ever smaller arteries, finally terminating in tiny twigs called capillaries. It is through the walls of the capillaries that the blood finally presents its gift of oxygen to the tissues. The venous system then collects the oxygen-depleted blood from the capillaries, eventually delivering it to the right ventricle of the heart, from where it will be sent to the lungs to become supplied with oxygen again. During the lifetime of a typical healthy eighty-year-old person, the heart will flawlessly perform its complicated pumping action, the heartbeat, more than three billion times. It is through this continuously cycling process that the body's never-ending requirement for oxygen is met.

In Tetralogy of Fallot, normal formation of cardiac anatomy goes awry during early embryonic development of the fetus. Tetralogy refers to the occurrence of four structural defects which constitute the complex malady. Besides a ventricular septal defect (a hole in the septum which separates the two ventricles) and stenosis (narrowing) of the pulmonic valve, the right ventricle is enlarged, and the aorta's connection to the left ventricle is misplaced. Because of this particular configuration of the abnormalities, a portion of the venous blood flows directly from the right to the left ventricle, bypassing the lungs altogether. From there it is pumped to the tissues, deprived of its usual content of oxygen. This detour is called shunting. In its diminished state this diverted blood is unable to provide the level of oxygen which nature intended for the body's tissues.

When Steve was a child, youngsters born with the Tetralogy defect could not run and play as normal children around them did, because their breath quickly failed them. Nor did they grow properly. In the first five years of his life, Stevie remained thin, his weight well below the normal range on the growth charts.

Some Tetralogy children develop the "blue baby syndrome," particularly if the shunting is severe. Stevie was one of these.

It is a December day in 1954, the dull, cold afternoon light already beginning to fade into darker shades of the approaching evening. We boys are dressed for outside winter play. Stevie is bundled in the green parka with the pointed hood that I remember so well. The drawstrings of the hood pulled tight, Stevie's small face peers out through its furry frame. Pete is pulling Stevie across the yard through ankle deep snow on the American Flyer sled that he was given as a Christmas present the year before. I am pushing, both hands on Stevie's back. When we reach the sidewalk I become aware of a change in Stevie. I begin to feel his labored breathing through the parka. Now I hear it, too. He is beginning to pant. "Pete," I shout, "hold up!" Pete slows, stops. I race around the side of the sled, and sure enough, Stevie is working hard. His eyes have that glassy, unfocused look, and he has turned a dusky grey-blue. Pete helps me get Stevie off the sled and onto his feet, and then, my hands on his shoulders, I push him downward into a squat, carefully, so that he does not lose his balance. Soon he relaxes and pinks up. Pete is already running home to get Mom or Dad.

We three brothers called these episodes "puffing." Stevie would unpredictably and suddenly turn blue (the medical term for this is cyanosis) and become short of breath. He was not sufficiently oxygenating his blood when this happened, and his organs and tissues were crying out in protest. Stevie's puffing didn't seem to be related to any particular type of activity or exertion. Most of the time the episodes could be magically relieved by his assuming a squatting posture. When Stevie went outside to play in the yard, it was a hard and fast rule that he always went out with two brothers; in case he started puffing, one of us would force him into a squat and remain with him while the other ran home for help.

The Race to Still a Beating Heart

The modern era of cardiac surgery began during World War II with the American surgeon Dwight Harkin. Following his research studies on dogs, Harkin, an officer in the Army Medical Corps, was able to successfully remove bullets and shrapnel from the hearts of about 100 American soldiers without a single fatality. Before this, most surgeons thought that operating on the heart would never be possible.

Following Harkin's experience, surgeons began to develop techniques to alleviate the consequences of certain cardiac abnormalities by operating on the closed heart and the great vessels around it. Perhaps the best known example of this palliative approach was the Blalock-Taussig shunt, a procedure developed in 1944 to improve the oxygenation of blood in patients with cyanotic heart disease. The procedure was first used in children with Tetralogy of Fallot. There have been modern updates to the procedure, but in its original version, the surgeon would simply isolate a main branch of the aorta (usually the subclavian artery) and connect it to a branch of the pulmonary artery, thus redirecting the patient's insufficiently oxygenated blood to the pulmonary circulation for another pass. But these operations were not curative: their goal was to relieve symptoms. Patients who were operated on often felt better for a while and sometimes even lived longer, but eventually they died when the temporary improvements gained through these procedures finally yielded to the inevitable progression of the underlying pathophysiologic abnormalities.

In the early 1950s few surgeons were tackling the problem of operating *inside* the heart. To perform repairs inside the heart itself, a quiet and dry operating field, free of currents of flowing blood, is needed. One might compare operating on a beating heart to trying to repair a broken automobile transmission while the car is moving. Delicate, complicated procedures are simply not possible. The heart has to be stilled. But how to do this without interrupting the flow of oxygenated blood to the patient's tissues, particularly the brain, which begins to die a mere four minutes after its supply of oxygen is interrupted?

Practicing on dogs, John Gibbon, a professor of surgery at Jefferson Medical College in Philadelphia, had labored for more than ten years to develop a machine that would provide cardiopulmonary bypass during surgery. In March 1953, he finally took his machine from the laboratory to the operating room. His first attempt at an operation inside a human heart while using his spinet piano-sized heart-lung bypass machine resulted in the death of a one-year-old child. The patient died not because of the failure of Gibbon's apparatus, but because the pre-operative diagnosis had been incorrect. His next patient, an eighteen-year-old woman, survived. In his third and fourth operations, two girls, both five years of age, succumbed. Gibbon called a halt to the further use of his machine and made no more attempts.

At about this time, at the University of Minnesota Medical School in Minneapolis, a young surgeon, C. Walton Lillehei, was also ready to move his experiments with extracorporeal circulation from the dog labs to clinical practice. He had developed a novel approach to the problem of providing cardiopulmonary support during heart surgery. For him, the "machine" was to be another human being, one of the patient's parents. Lillehei called his method "controlled cross-circulation."

On March 26, 1954, Gregory Glidden, a sickly thirteen-month-old child from the Iron Range town of Hibbing, Minnesota, was taken to the operating room, where Lillehei's team was waiting. Minutes later his donor father was wheeled in on a gurney. After each of them was anesthetized, catheters were placed in Gregory's superior vena cava and aorta, and in the femoral artery and vein of his father. A pump was interposed between the two patients in order to maintain precise control over the flow of blood. Blood was routed from Gregory's caval vein to the femoral vein of his father. From there it passed to the paternal heart, where it was pumped into the lungs and oxygenated. The arterial oxygen-rich blood was then returned to Gregory's aorta from the femoral artery of his father. In the nineteen minutes that Gregory was receiving oxygen-rich blood from his father, Lillehei accomplished the world's first repair of a ventricular septal defect. Gregory died of post-operative pneumonia two weeks later. His death was devastating to Lillehei, but from a technical and surgical standpoint the operation had been a success. The door to intra-cardiac surgery had been opened and the surgeon's foot was firmly in the door. Doctors now knew that support of the patient's physiologic needs during exposure of the internal structures of the heart was possible. In the mid-1950s Lillhei and his team performed forty-four subsequent open heart surgeries using this technique, but with forty percent intra- or post-operative mortality.

* * *

Stevie grew from a toddler to a towheaded little boy. He played with us, but he would tire easily. His puffing spells, always unpredictable, were becoming more frequent as he grew into his pre-school years. They became a source of embarrassment for him. "Once we were playing in the snow," Steve recollects. "We were having a snowball fight in the Salmens' back yard, and at some point I did my squatting because I got short of breath. You guys were taught to put me in a squat, which would usually make me breathe easier, and to get Mom when I had those spells. I remember her coming then and dragging me away on a sled in the middle of that fight, and I didn't want to leave. I remember often looking out of the living room window at other neighborhood kids playing outside, especially in the winter, wishing that I could be out there with them."

Sometimes after a spell had subsided, Stevie would remain tired and drained, and at these times our parents would have him inhale oxygen for a while, administered through a face mask. Here was another embarrassment for him: the twice weekly appearance at our house on Highland Parkway of the "oxygen truck." Stevie anticipated its arrival because Mom would announce, "The oxygen truck is coming today." The panel truck that arrived to deliver the large, heavy, green cylinders was plainly marked. He wished it would come at night, so that his friends wouldn't see it. "I just didn't want to be different," he recalls.

The rules for us brothers were simple: We were not allowed to tease Stevie, chase him, or otherwise upset him. We occasionally broke these rules, of course, but for the most part we were careful with him so as not to cause more puffing, since those spells could be frightening. Besides, none of us wished to upset Mom or provoke a stern, reproving scolding from Dad.

Weekends were for haircuts given by Dad on Saturday mornings, and sometimes for Sunday family outings after Mass and lunch. Pete recalls one such Sunday afternoon when Steve was about four years old. Mom and Dad had brought us to an amusement park. Our favorite ride there was the bumper cars. After fares were paid for Stevie, Tom, and me, and everyone was strapped in securely, the operator threw the switch. Immediately, poles sparking off the overhead electrical grid, the cars began to lurch around the rink ramming into each other, each collision provoking shrieks of laughter. As we stood behind the railing watching the action, Mom remarked to Pete, "Why look at Stevie. He's like a little mouse out there."

We boys had regular medical visits to our pediatrician in his downtown St. Paul office. Dr. Charles Steinberg was a handsome man with a head of fine, silver-grey hair and a pencil-thin moustache; well into his fifties he still cut a trim figure. He had a gravel-toned voice and always seemed to have a lit cigarette in his hand. My parents, especially my mother, trusted his judgment completely, and their faith in him was not limited to medical matters. Over the years he became a font of moral authority and wisdom for our family. I am certain that somehow his presence in our family life influenced my choice of career, and perhaps Steve's as well. He also influenced our lives in countless smaller ways. When I was about nine years old, my parents bought our first television, a black and white Magnavox. We kids soon learned that in addition to early westerns such as *Hopalong Cassidy* and the *Lone Ranger*, other intriguing programs forbidden to us children by parental order were becoming popular. We were most curious about one of these newer programs, called *Dragnet*. Although our friends across the street excitedly described Sergeant Joe Friday and his sleuthing, we were not allowed to watch this series because its theme was crime. Finally, after weeks of complaining and pleading,

Mom agreed to call Dr. Steinberg and ask him whether we should be allowed to watch the show. After prudent reflection, he advised her that since there was no explicit depiction of violence in *Dragnet,* and since the bad guys inevitably were caught and punished, there was no harm in our watching it. We had won the day! We were ecstatic.

* * *

Meanwhile, Lillehei was becoming the darling of the press and a star in the medical world. His surgery using controlled cross-circulation was brilliant and daring, and his cures were stunning. Children with no future were being discharged from the hospital to a normal childhood and presumably a normal life expectancy.

As my parents read these stories, their hopes rose. Every three months they would drive Steve to his appointment with the pediatric cardiologist at the Variety Club Heart Hospital. Steve doesn't recall much about visits. He only remembers the exercise treadmill and other physiologic testing.

I imagine Mom and Dad sitting in the waiting room with Steve between them, wondering if this time he would be referred to Lillehei's program. But in the end, the cardiologist and his colleagues decided against offering Steve an attempt at surgical correction because, in addition to his Tetralogy of Fallot, he had severe narrowing of the left pulmonary artery and consequently had an underdeveloped left lung. In their judgment the odds against Steve surviving the operation were prohibitively high. "What should we do?" Mom asked the cardiologist in near desperation as she and Dad dressed Stevie, preparing to leave his office. "Bring him back when he turns black. Then, maybe, we'll see." was the answer. It appeared that Stevie would have little chance for a curative operation at the University.

Those were surely difficult days for Mom and Dad, knowing as they did that Stevie had virtually no chance of reaching his teenage years, and that catastrophe could befall him at any moment. Tom and I had little awareness of their discouragement and growing desperation.

Pete, however, remembers their distress clearly: "Mom and Dad were constantly worried about Steve. He was always on their minds.

They were stressed, and both tried to hide it, Dad in particular. He didn't want us kids to see his hurt and worry. Mom was less successful at hiding her pain. I remember thinking that Mom had turned into somebody different after Steve was born. I was eight years old when he came along. Early, I remember her being fun-loving, laughing a lot. She developed a serious side after he arrived. She became crabby much of the time. I didn't know why at first, but I eventually figured it out. It was Steve. It was just something we had to accept. She had a tremendous amount of stress. Dad was more stoic. He was the steady one, the rock. But he was gone a lot. Communication in the early fifties was not what it is today, and when he was on the road Mom was left alone with her worries about Steve and the stress of raising four boys."

One evening at dinner early in 1953, my parents announced that we would make a family pilgrimage to pray for a miracle to spare Stevie's life. We would travel to the shrine of Sainte Anne de Beaupré in Québec Province. This sanctuary, located about thirty miles east of Québec City, is situated on a hillside that slopes down to the St. Lawrence River. It is North America's oldest and most prominent shrine east of the Mississippi. When we arrived there in the summer of 1953, St. Anne had been granting miraculous relief of pilgrims' physical ailments for nearly three hundred years.

On a warm June morning that year, the six of us stuffed ourselves and our suitcases into the family car, a lime-green 1953 Buick, and began the several-day drive to the Canadian shrine. To keep expenses down our meals were mostly picnics—breakfast, lunch, and dinner. Most of those were not pleasant affairs. We endured the rain picnic and the ant picnic. The caterpillar picnic, when dozens of larvae dropped from the overhanging tree branches down our backs, onto our sandwiches, and into our drinks, is captured on grainy eight-millimeter film, probably taken by Dad using Uncle Carl's Bell & Howell wind-up home-movie camera. At night we slept in three-bed rooms in cheap motels. Our trip in the car was a running scene of giggling, teasing, crying, and sleeping as the pastoral scenery swept by the car windows, mostly unnoticed by us boys. Every afternoon about four o'clock our parents rewarded each of us with one small plastic toy for good behavior. I remember being given a plastic pistol and a red car with black wheels. Pete and Tom often fought with each other in the back seat, eleven-year-old Pete taunting his younger brother, "The big, bad wolf will come and eat you up!" On these days neither Pete nor his victim received a toy.

I recall little of our visit to the site itself. I only know that Mom climbed the steps to the shrine on her knees and made a vow to St. Anne never to eat chocolate again if Steve were spared. Her determination to find a cure for him was like iron.

It was our custom each Memorial Day to visit Calvary Cemetery as a family, to pray briefly at the graves of Mom's parents and her sister, Ida. In 1955, Grandma, Dad's mother, accompanied us to the grave site. Dad's father was not there. No one knew his whereabouts. Grandma threw him out for his boozing when Dad was six years old. At the cemetery, we three boys trailed our parents, Dad leading the way, pulling Steve in a red wagon down the elm-shaded path. I noticed that Mom was quietly crying as we ambled along, but I kept silent. Later that evening when we were at home, I asked Dad why Mom was crying. "Because she thinks we'll be visiting Stevie's grave next year," he replied.

* * *

At the same time that C. Walton Lillehei was producing groundbreaking innovations in cardiac surgery at the University of Minnesota, another young surgeon at the Mayo Clinic in Rochester was addressing the problem of heart-lung bypass by resurrecting an old idea. John W. Kirklin was a thirty-eight-year-old staff surgeon at the Clinic. He and his team had been refining the boxy heart-lung bypass machine of John Gibbon. Because of Lillehei's spectacular successes at the University, the Mayo surgeon was under pressure to abandon his machine in favor of his colleague's controlled cross-circulation. But Kirklin resisted, foreseeing the limitations of broad applicability of the controlled cross-circulation method. "Imagine," one critic observed, "a surgery with a potential for 200% mortality—both the patient and donor!" Kirklin was confident that he and his team had developed a superior and a safer technology.

For several years, Kirklin had been preoccupied with the possibility of repairing previously uncorrectable congenital heart defects. There must be some way to meet the patient's oxygen and perfusion requirements while the heart was paralyzed and cleared of blood, he thought. Later in his career he related how he and his fellow surgical residents would sit around for hours at night drawing diagrams of possible repairs for various defects, including Tetralogy of Fallot, if only they could get inside the heart.

In 1952 Kirklin and a few colleagues visited three academic medical centers which had previously attempted to develop a heart-lung bypass machine. None was actively pursuing its research or development at the time. Of the three, the group thought that the Jefferson Medical College's Gibbon-IBM pump oxygenator was most promising. Supported by IBM chairman Thomas J. Watson, Gibbon had designed a system in which blood was oxygenated by passing a thin film of it over a membrane in an oxygen-rich atmosphere.

Negotiations between the Mayo Clinic and Jefferson Medical College ensued and resulted in delivery of the design plans for the Gibbon-IBM pump to Mayo. Kirklin rapidly assembled a team of experts that included pediatric and adult cardiologists, mechanical engineers, a renowned cardiac pathologist, a physiologist, and an anesthesiologist, all of whom participated in the redesign effort. After many months, the Gibbon machine emerged from the Mayo Clinic's engineering shops as the Mayo-Gibbon heart-lung bypass machine. It was now ready for the dogs.

Kirklin spent the next two and a half years operating day and night inside canine hearts, continually modifying and refining the machine. In early 1955 he was finally ready to apply the technology to humans. He received Mayo's backing to proceed with a series of five patients (later this was expanded to eight), and anticipated that a number of them might not survive the operation. Nonetheless, so confident was he in the machine's technology and so certain of its potential benefits, that he told each patient's family that even if he lost several of his first patients, he would proceed to operate on the rest.

The first surgery was closure of a ventricular septal defect, performed in May 1955 by Kirklin at Rochester Methodist Hospital. The operation was a success, and the patient, a five-and-a-half-year-old child, left the hospital after ten days. Seven additional patients subsequently underwent open heart surgery while being supported on the Mayo-Gibbon cardiopulmonary bypass machine. Of those first eight patients, four died during surgery or post-operatively. From this experience came the world's first medical publication reporting the use of mechanical cardiopulmonary support on a group of open heart patients.

At about the same time that Kirklin was conducting his clinical work on the pump, Lillehei abandoned his technique of controlled cross-circulation at the University of Minnesota. Instead, he concentrated on his own cardiopulmonary bypass machine, which he had been refining in his laboratory, assisted by his colleague, Richard De-Wall. They called their machine a bubble pump oxygenator. Instead of a Mayo-Gibbon type of membrane for oxygenating the blood, they used a system which created bubbles by injecting fine streams of oxygen into the blood.

Reflecting on this era many years later, the eminent Stanford cardiac surgeon Norman Shumway said, "There for a shining moment, the only institutions in the world where one could go for open heart surgery were 90 miles apart, at the Mayo Clinic and the University of Minnesota."

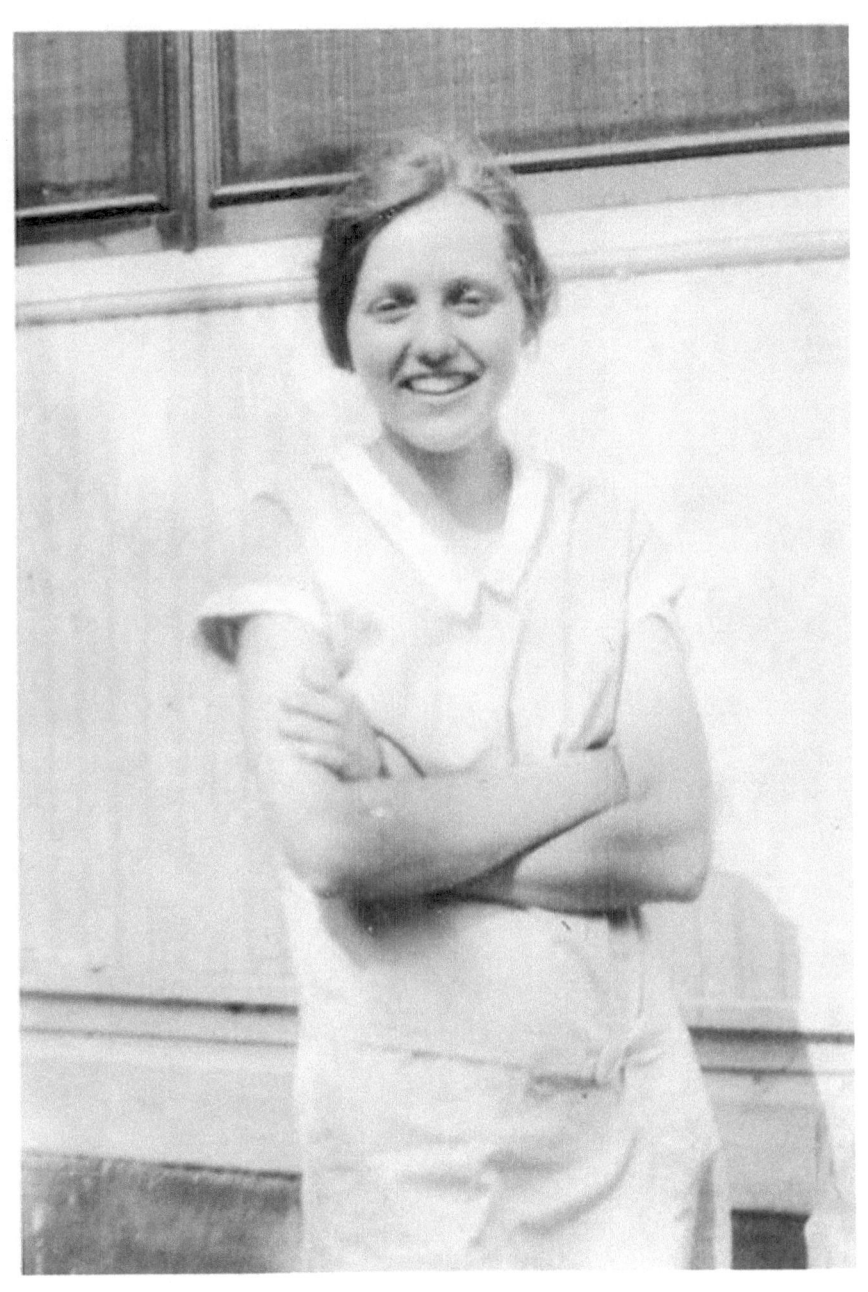

Mom at age 28

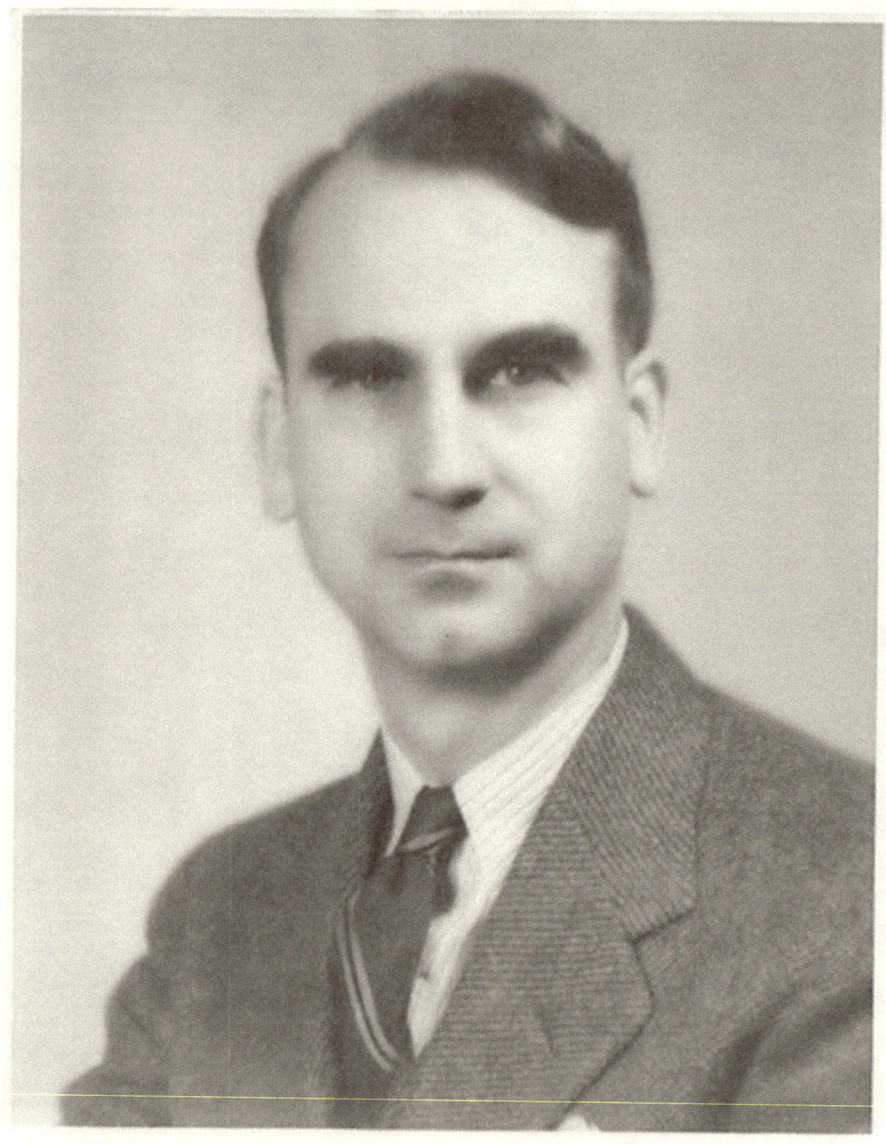

Dad in his early 30s

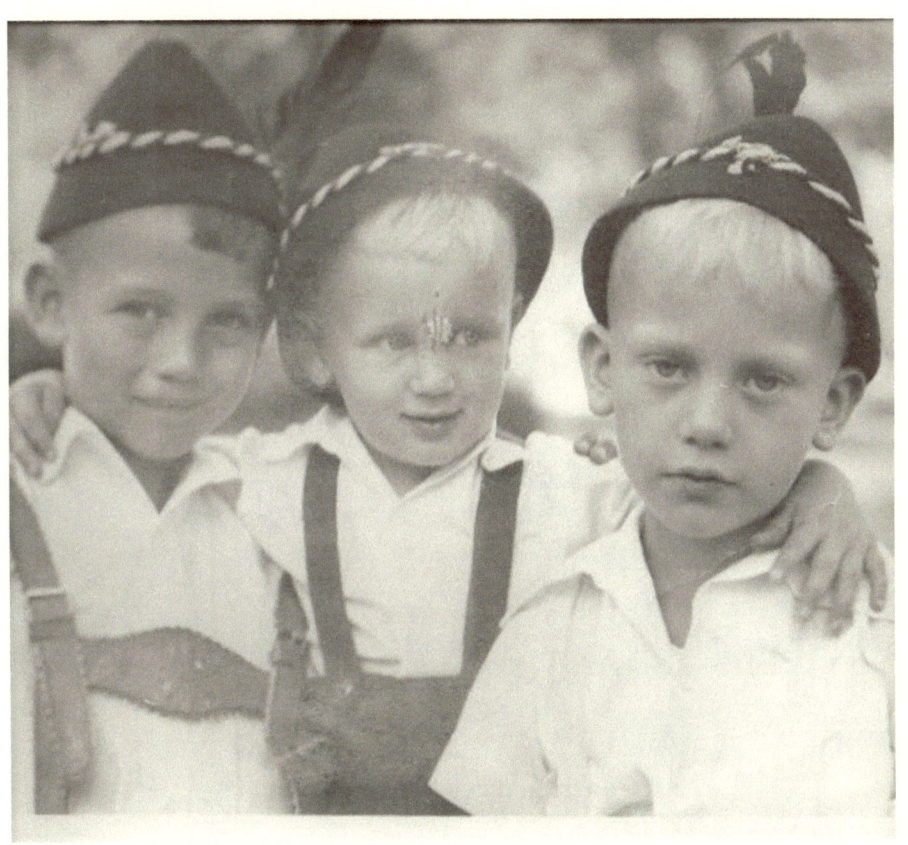

Pete, Tom, and Mike before Stevie arrived

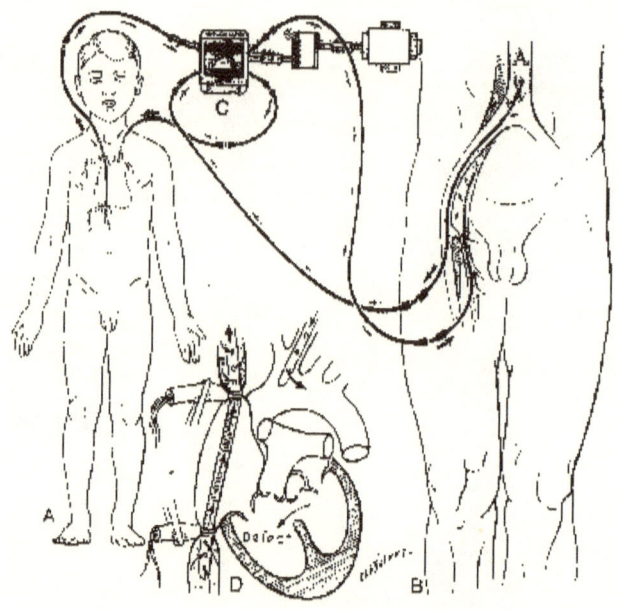

Controlled cross-circulation

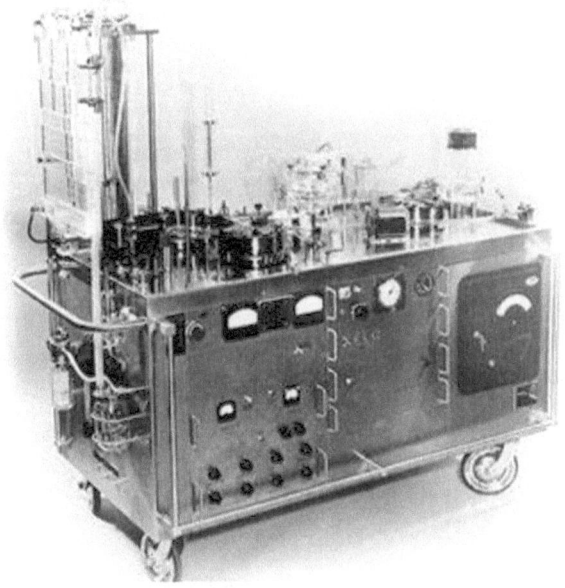

Mayo-Gibbon heart-lung bypass machine

Michael Carl Brabeck

Proceedings of the

STAFF MEETINGS OF THE MAYO CLINIC

Published Fortnightly for the Information of the Members of the Staff and the Fellows of the Mayo Foundation for Medical Education and Research

Volume 30   ROCHESTER, MINNESOTA, WEDNESDAY, MAY 18, 1955   Number 10

CONTENTS

Kirklin's landmark 1955 publication

22

December 1956:

"It is probably superfluous to tell you that Stevie is in A-1 shape this winter. He's leading a new life, and still now and then refers to the fact that Dr. Kirklin's 'operation' (sic) makes all this possible for him.

Again, may we express our gratitude to you? We never can forget!"

December 1959

"Stevie is fine. We never fail to remember that if it weren't for the dedication of men like you, we wouldn't have a healthy boy, such as Stephen is today!"

December 1960

"Stevie continues to do well. We'll never forget how well you took care of him!"

December 1961

"Stevie is fine. We'll see you next spring!"

Christmas Messages to Dr. Kirklin from George and Marie Brabeck

Salvation

Mom and Dad arrived with Stevie at the Mayo Clinic in Rochester in late September 1955, two weeks after Mom had heard Dr. Kirklin describe his experimental surgery on the *Medical Horizons* program. In Rochester there was hope after rejection at the University of Minnesota. Hope lay in the heritage of innovation at the Mayo Clinic, and in the determination and confidence of the young surgeon directing Mayo's open heart initiative.

I recently asked Steve if he remembered Dr. Kirklin on that first visit. Steve recalls him clearly. "He had incredible piercing eyes. Even as a five-year-old kid, those eyes got your attention. He was neither friendly nor unfriendly, but it was as if he were looking right into you through his wire-rimmed spectacles. He had very angular features, with a thin, pointed, nose. Everything was very thin about him. He had a serious demeanor."

Stevie carried his floppy, worn Teddy bear into the consultation room that morning. Before he and the three adults sat down, Dr. Kirklin shook Stevie's hand and asked, "What's his name?" Thinking that the doctor was inquiring about the name of his dad, Stevie replied, "George." So for the rest of the hour Dr. Kirklin referred to the Teddy bear as "George." Stevie realized that a mistake had been made, but he had no idea how to correct it, so for that morning the Teddy's name remained George.

Kirklin told my parents what they already knew from watching the *Medical Horizons* program: that he and his colleagues had completed a series of eight open heart operations using their heart-lung bypass machine, and that four of their eight patients had died. Nonetheless, Kirklin assured them that the team's sophistication and the performance of the machine were improving with each case. Kirklin's confidence was growing. He was seeking more patients. As the consultation neared its end, he informed my parents that he would accept Stevie as a patient, which meant that despite Stevie's underdeveloped left pulmonary artery and lung, Kirklin would attempt to repair his Tetralogy of Fallot.

The date for Stevie's operation was set for December 5, 1955, and the inevitable waiting began. Dad and Mom restricted Stevie's activities and exertions even more tightly than before. In November there were several appointments at the Mayo Clinic for pre-operative testing. We boys accompanied Stevie and our parents on a few of those trips. When overnights were necessary we would stay at the Kahler Hotel, directly across West Center Street from Rochester Methodist, where the surgery would be performed. Sometimes there would be an extra treat for us. Dad took Tom one evening to see Audie Murphy in *To Hell and Back*. On another occasion Mom and Dad took Stevie to see *Moby Dick*, starring Gregory Peck.

Stevie, the focus of those visits and days, had little understanding at the time of what was planned for him. He can only recall Mom saying that Dr. Kirklin was going to make him better: "When you're five years old, it's your parents who control the shots. You're just living in the moment from hour to hour, and you're not into worrying about the future. Your brain just doesn't work that way at age five years. So I have no memory of trying to understand or worrying, because the thoughts simply weren't there."

Steve began to feel special. On each of these visits to the Clinic he was given an early Christmas present. One time it was a Candy Land board game. He received a bag of building blocks on another visit. When I asked Steve if he ever thought about dying during those days, he answered with a simple "no." As far as he was concerned, he was just a kid getting a lot of very nice attention, especially since most of the time his brothers had to stay back at home in St. Paul, minded by Tante Ida.

For Pete, Tom, and me, Tante Ida was our most unpleasant memory of this period. She stayed with us whenever Mom, Dad, and Stevie needed to be in Rochester. She was stern and gloomy, and we felt that she was overly strict with us. She accused us on more than one occasion of pocketing loose change from Dad's top dresser drawer. Overnights with our friends were not permitted. Tom's only favorable recollection of all our time with her is the sticky buns she used to make for us most mornings before school. Tante Ida had emigrated from Germany many years before. She had been a maid in some of St. Paul's finest mansions, where her husband, Onkel Ernst, who was Swiss, worked as chief butler. We were always glad when Onkel Ernst came to visit. Unlike her, he was cheerful and jokey, and he had the longest earlobes we had ever seen.

At eight o'clock in the morning on December 5, a nurse came to Stevie's hospital room to take him to the operating theater. He remembers Mom and Dad standing on the right side of the gurney on which he was sitting. He's not sure any more, but thinks that Mom was trying to hide her tears. They walked beside him for a short distance down the hall, then were not allowed to proceed farther. "And then I rolled off alone with the nurse who was soothing me," he recalls.

Once in the operating room, Stevie was lifted from the gurney to operating table, and presently someone asked him to count the lights over the table, which were arranged in a circle on the ceiling. A rubber mask was placed over his face, and he felt frustrated because he could no longer see to count the lights. Moreover, the intense smell of the Neoprene rubber was noxious, and Stevie felt a rising panic. Steve wonders to this day if his claustrophobic tendencies result from the experience of that anesthesia mask.

Just before ten o'clock that morning, an announcement was made over the public address system at St. Leo the Great, the parochial grade school in St. Paul that we Brabeck boys attended. I was in sixth grade at the time, Pete was in eighth, and Tom in third. We heard the voice of the school principal, Sister James Marie, directing that all activity stop for a period of two minutes, and that we pray for the success of the surgery of "little Stevie Brabeck with a hole in his heart, who is being operated on at this moment."

Beginning the operation, Dr. Kirklin first made a clamshell incision, which is a horizontal cut running the entire breadth of the chest just below the nipple line. This allowed the entire upper chest to be lifted to expose the heart. (The clamshell incision is rarely if ever used today in modern cardiac surgery.) Stevie's circulatory system was then attached to the Mayo-Gibbon cardiopulmonary bypass machine via a series of tubes. Soon the pump was turned on and began to supply his anesthetized body with freshly oxygenated blood. Next his heart was chemically paralyzed. An hour later, Dr. Kirklin and his team had patched the ventricular septal defect and repaired his stenotic pulmonary valve, corrections that would last Steve for more than fifty years.

Stevie's surgery went well. There was no complication, and upon removal from the life-supporting heart-lung bypass apparatus, his heart resumed its normal function. The post-operative recuperation, however, was not so easy for the little patient.

Stevie was assigned a special duty nurse, Miss Joan Grevsted. She was a smallish woman, a redhead with a deep, resonant, smoker's voice, whom Stevie regarded as "my best buddy" during his period of recuperation. She looked after him daily and called him "the best little boy on the seven seas." Mom and Dad were with Steve every day as well, of course, and thus began a friendship between them and Miss Grevsted that continued for many years.

Steve recounts, "I remember how parched I was post-op. I was on fluid restriction. I was in an oxygen tent, where I slept at night and sat during the day. There were these plastic see-through flaps, and I'd be sitting on the inside on my bed, looking out at everyone else who was on the outside. I was so damned thirsty. Humidified oxygen came from a vent somewhere, and there was a condenser above my head, slowly dripping water. I remember looking up and trying to catch those drops of water on my tongue.

"Every day a nurse came to give me a penicillin shot—two shots in fact, one of which was penicillin. I don't know what the other was. They really hurt, and I didn't like it at all. I hated seeing that door open in the morning, and would let loose and scream each morning when they came in with those syringes.

"I remember the day they removed my chest tubes as clearly as if they had come out yesterday. It wasn't fun. The surgeon who came in to take them out—I don't remember his name—had black curly hair. He said that it was going to hurt a little bit, which scared the heck out of me. By that time I had been getting those daily shots, so I was well programmed to be terrified of more pain. And did it hurt! I screamed when they pulled them out, nurses on each side of me holding my arms down. It was a bloody mess. I remember looking down and seeing all the blood."

Two weeks after his surgery, Stevie left the hospital and returned to St. Paul with Mom and Dad. Life slowly returned to normal for him and our family—mostly. In the winter after his surgery, Stevie was still not allowed to walk to school. He was driven to St. Leo's, where he would remain inside the warm car until the bell rang and school doors opened to admit the pupils. Stevie felt humiliated by having to stay in the car with his mom while his friends dashed about on the playground. But our parents tried to make his life as normal as possible. According to Steve, "When I look back today on that time after my surgery, they worked hard on not letting me be different from the other kids. I think that a lot of parents who had just had their five-year-old child go through a new, experimental, life-saving operation, would hover over that kid for a few years. Not Mom or Dad, no way. In the spring, Mayo pronounced me healthy and fit, and I don't remember any more restrictions after that. My life at home and at school was entirely normal after that winter, and through the rest of grade school, high school, and college."

Stevie's memories of his early childhood and surgery at age five years faded with the advance of puberty and adolescence. Occasionally he'd be standing in the bathroom brushing his teeth before bed, and Dad would comment on the railroad tracks going across his chest. After a while that scar was the only reminder he had of what he'd gone through.

Growing up

Stevie gradually morphed into Steve, and after his sixteenth birthday, his annual checkups at the Mayo Clinic ceased. He did not return to Mayo again for more than forty-one years.

When Steve was in his early twenties, Mom sat down with him one afternoon and told him that she thought the time had come that she could be released from her promise to St. Anne. She began to eat chocolates again, and from that time on, Steve's congenital heart disease and his rescue from it receded into our family history and lore, and remained only as a distant memory.

Steve attended St. Thomas College (now the University of St. Thomas), a small Catholic liberal arts college in St. Paul, while living at home with Mom and Dad. He was attracted to life sciences and chose to major in biology. Early in his college career, he became aware that he liked to work with people. It would seem that he had set out from the beginning to become a physician. But he maintains that his choice of career was more conditional than planned. He says that, in some small way, it was influenced by my being in medical school while he was in college. Steve recalls me coming home from classes at the University of Minnesota and from work at the hospital with new interests and a new jargon, which he found intriguing. He decided to apply to medical school himself. He received his MD degree from the University of Minnesota in 1976, six years after I received mine.

Cardiology was a different story. Nearly everyone, when they hear the story of Steve's congenital heart disease and cure, assumes that he became a cardiologist because of his personal history. While that probably had some impact on his decision, Steve maintains that it was not central. Because he does not wish to disappoint those hoping for a more romantic explanation, Steve does not often reveal the real reason behind his choice, which he disclosed to me in a recent conversation:

"Cardiology scared the hell out of me. In my internship year I was intimidated by it. When someone comes in with an acute heart problem, you've got *golden minutes* to make an accurate diagnosis and institute the correct therapy, and in some cases only golden seconds. You don't have an hour for sure, which you do in most other situations in internal medicine. If you're not right on your toes, disaster may occur. That's scary as hell and I just didn't like it. I used to shudder when a cardiac case came in. I would always think, what if I screw this up? I knew that this fear would haunt me my entire professional career, and I said to myself that I've got a long career ahead of me, and if I want to be a competent internist, I can't continue this way. Finally I got to the point where I said, screw it. The way to take care of a problem is to face it head on, and for me, the solution was to immerse myself in it. I had to recognize the elephant in the room and confront it. That's why I did the fellowship in cardiology, so that I'd be thrown into the fray and become immune to that terror. The first year of fellowship for me was like a feeding frenzy of learning. I quickly came to love the field."

Because Marie Brabeck and Peg Maykoski were close friends, Steve probably encountered Peg's daughter, Lisi, during his childhood at occasional gatherings of their two families. An old undated photo shows young children from both families, including Steve and Lisi, sitting around a picnic table in a park. But Steve has no memories of these occasions.

His first clear recollection of Lisi is in a college sociology class in which they were both enrolled at the College of St. Catherine, a women's college in St. Paul known locally as St. Kate's, and co-institutional with St. Thomas College. At that time Lisi had been in an apparently committed relationship for four years with a young man who was attending the University of Notre Dame. Both of their families expected them to marry. After class one day, a mutual friend introduced Steve to Lisi. Steve, who was living at home at the time, remembers telling Mom that evening, "You'll never guess who I met today in my sociology class. I met Lisi Maykoski."

Steve and Lisi hung around with a group of mutual college buddies. They studied together, often while watching *Star Trek*, and went out for good times as a group. Steve and Lisi became friends, but early on, romantic interest was absent.

One day in early 1972, Mom gave Steve two tickets to an evening performance of Bach arias at St. Kate's, where she had received her master's degree in music nearly forty years before. Not wanting to disappoint her, Steve decided to attend the performance, and he accepted the tickets. Steve describes himself as being "between relationships" at that time, and says he couldn't find anyone to accompany him that evening. As Lisi laughingly tells the story, Steve telephoned her to explain that he'd been unable to get a date for the Bach concert, and would she like to go? Lisi still maintains that she has no idea why she accepted the invitation when put that way. But she went with him anyway, and they left the performance at the intermission. They laughed about how boring it had been, and felt guilty pleasure in leaving early. After a midnight meal in a small Italian restaurant in the neighborhood, they bid each other good night, but each was beginning to think that there might be something more to their relationship than just being good friends.

Another time that Steve thought there might be a growing attraction between them was one winter night at St. Kate's. He had arrived on the campus in a car with several friends. Lisi was walking outside with a couple of her girlfriends, saw them pull up, and began to laugh as he opened the car door. She reached down, made some quick snowballs and threw them at Steve while he was still in the car, but only at Steve. He remembers thinking, "Hmm…!"

Steve recalls their first kiss: "We're standing there, and she kissed me with her eyes wide open. I'd never kissed a girl whose eyes were staring at me while I was kissing her. As we were kissing, I remember thinking, this is Aunt Peg's daughter! It was a creepy, almost incestuous feeling."

The two grew closer. But Lisi still hadn't broken off with her boyfriend at Notre Dame, and Steve became increasingly uncomfortable. He continues, "So we finally had a talk. I said to her that we can't go on this way, you've got to make a choice. It's got to be one or the other of us, but not both any more. I know you care a lot about Dave, and it's not fair to him or me. So it's over until you make a choice. I remember us slowly walking and talking in thick fog down by the Ford's Twin Cities Assembly Plant near Hidden Falls. She had driven us down there in her old Vega. When there was no more to be said, I asked her to leave me there. I said I'd walk home. I remember seeing her drive off, disappearing into that fog, and I felt just miserable. It was the loneliest night of my life.

"For two weeks I heard nothing from her. Then one afternoon I was standing with Dad, who was roasting a chicken for dinner on the rotisserie in the garage. Suddenly I'm aware of him looking at something over my shoulder. He was watching a woman on a bicycle peddling furiously down Highland Parkway. And then I heard the bicycle hit the pavement with a crash. It was Lisi. She was running up the driveway, and she grabbed me. Dad realized that he should exit the scene, and he did, quickly. We hugged. She was crying. She had made her choice."

Steve decided to propose marriage to Lisi in late 1974, but before asking her to marry him, he needed to revisit an old issue. Steve felt he had to know, with as much certainty as possible, if he might have a limited future. Until then he had assumed, with the blind confidence of healthy and exuberant youth, that he was immortal, or at least that he had been fixed for good. But now he did not want to offer Lisi the prospect of committing to a man with poor odds for long-term survival.

At about this time, Steve had two unexplained near-fainting episodes. These, and his need for a realistic assessment of his health prospects, prompted him to seek consultation at the University's Student Health Service. From there he was referred to the Variety Club Heart Hospital, the site of his rejection in early 1955. His underwent cardiac catheterization, performed by Dr. Yang Wang, a noted pediatric cardiologist, and Dr. Kurt Amplatz, the Austrian radiologist renowned for his inventions of vascular and intra-cardiac radiologic devices. They performed electrophysiologic and hemodymanic studies, and the news was good. Steve learned that he had pulmonic insufficiency (an absent or nonfunctional pulmonary valve), the significance of which was not then fully understood or appreciated. Everything else looked fine.

I was a medical resident at the University at the time and visited Steve in his hospital room soon after the procedure. He was lying flat on his hospital bed with a pressure dressing over his groin. He grinned and told me that he could now proceed.

Steve asked Lisi to marry him on April 13, 1975, at a small Mississippi riverfront bar & grill on St. Anthony Main. Pracna on Main is the oldest restaurant in Minneapolis. A waterfront institution, it is situated on one of the first streets built in the city, a cobblestone avenue lined on the landward side by antique nineteenth century red-brick buildings. Looking across the Mississsippi from Pracna's windows, one sees the skyline of downtown Minneapolis.

"I had no ring," Steve says, "but I asked her anyway, and she said yes. So there wasn't a burst of passion between us that suddenly ignited. It was a process of growth. Our relationship grew over time from friendship into romance, but the friendship has remained, and that has been the strength of our marriage. I married my best friend, and so did she."

The Cardiologist

Steve and Lisi were married in a small wedding ceremony at the Holy Family Catholic Church in Hillman, Minnesota, on August 23, 1975. On that day, Peg Maykoski, Mom's old friend whose telephone call led to Steve's cure at the Mayo Clinic twenty years earlier, became his mother-in-law.

After several years of practice as a general internist in Minnesota, and later as a cardiologist in New England, Steve and Lisi settled on the Monterey Peninsula in northern California. Lisi is now a school teacher. She has devoted her career to the education of children with special needs. Their own four children are now grown. The fifth, Ghion, whom they adopted as a four-year-old child from Ethiopia, is a teenager.

Steve, noted for his expertise in the treatment of heart failure, currently practices in a prominent group of heart and lung specialists located near his and Lisi's home. He holds a clinical faculty appointment at University of California San Francisco School of Medicine. Steve has been associated with the American Heart Association for over 15 years, serving as board member and as divisional and affiliate president. He is also serves on the board of the fledgling Adult Congenital Heart Association.

As a medical doctor myself for more than thirty-seven years, I understand the qualities that distinguish an ordinary from an excellent physician. Steve is the embodiment of these, and has long been a role model for me.

One of the attributes that makes Steve an exceptional physician is that he is a specialist in diseases of the heart who also has extensive experience in general (adult) internal medicine: he was a general internist for eight years, including a four-year stint as the sole Indian Health Service physician on the Red Lake Indian Reservation in northern Minnesota, before pursuing his training in cardiology. When you are Steve's patient, he will of course focus on your cardiac issues. But he will also consider other diseases or dysfunctional organ systems you may have, which may or may not directly relate to his specialty, and he will place his analysis of your heart problems in the context of you as a whole person. Not many physicians do this, and fewer do it so well.

Today Steve often encounters those cardiac emergencies which so terrified him earlier in his training. Not long ago I received the following e-mail from him:

Mike,

Today was one of those days that try docs' souls. It was one of those go-to-the-maker, test-your-mettle days. Scary as hell when it's going on, but exhilarating in its own way, and gives pause for reflection as it's winding down. I often feel that, although it's in a scaled down way, it must be similar to the process one feels who goes through battle.

This morning I was enjoying one of my partner's presentations on cardiac CT scans at grand rounds, when I was stat-paged to the ER. When I arrived, I was confronted with a 41-year-old lady *in extremis,* sitting bolt upright, a panicked look on her face, you know, the "My god, I think I'm going to die, *please* don't let me die" look. She was terrified and was hemoptysizing, dyspneic, constricted, in normotensive shock, with a stat echocardiogram showing an ejection fraction of ~5-10%. She was 34 weeks pregnant, mother of 5 kids at home. She probably had peripartum cardiomyopathy. We got her intubated, but couldn't oxygenate her even then. We shot her over to the ICU where the intensivist and I set up lines for hemodynamic monitoring, had the dobutamine, dopamine, Lasix infusions, etc, running, and she crashed further. She was losing her blood pressure, and he baby's heart rate fell to 30. There went our plans to stabilize her before surgery. Everyone was then called *stat*: the pediatrician, the obstetrician, cardiac anesthesia, and we rushed her to the OR. OB did the C-section in 6 minutes flat, while we put in an intra-aortic balloon pump, Swann Ganz catheter, and arterial lines. She was now on maximum doses of levophed, neosynephrine, and dopamine. Baby came out with low APGAR's, which immediately improved. With 1:1 pump augmentation, mom also started to improve. A little bladder sweat started to appear, then more. Tonight I have her off all pressors, on a 1:1 pump, nesiritide, dobutamine, and lasix infusions still running. We've got this as a result: augmented BP of 130, MAP 100, urine output 200/hr, pO2 330 torr on 40% FiO2 (up from 80 torr on 100%), cardiac index in high 2's, warm hands and feet, and good eye contact and communication with family. Finally, the day is nearly over. This is probably one of the best end-of-the-days I've experienced in my career. Before going home, I made a trip to the newborn unit, a place I had to ask directions to, since I hadn't been there before. There was a beautiful little guy, pink, moving, breathing on his own, looking around. Peds [pediatrics] says he's just fine. They don't expect any neurologic sequelae, and he should have a normal life. All I can say, 'two-fer's' are usually good, but this one is uncommonly so. From time to time it hits you how blessed we are to do what we do, doesn't it?

Lil' bro Steve

Steve's devotion to his patients' welfare embodies the essential principles of altruism and beneficence in the medical profession. He understands that the secret of patient care lies in caring about the patient. His partners at Cardio-Pulmonary Associates Medical Group, and of course his patients, have long known this about him.

Rejoicing, then Relapse

In May 2005, I received a telephone call from Lisi. She asked that my wife, Mary, and I set aside the first weekend in December: she was planning a dinner for Steve's family, friends, and colleagues to celebrate the fiftieth anniversary of his surgery at the Mayo Clinic. It was to be a surprise for Steve.

On Saturday afternoon of that December weekend, Pete, Tom, and I converged from the farthest points of the United States (including Alaska, where Pete was living at the time) to meet in a tavern in the center of Salinas, California. Mary was with us; Barbara, Tom's wife, had come as well. Mom's brother, Uncle Bill, who is a Catholic priest and former rector of the St. Paul Seminary, was in the group. He had flown in from St. Paul that morning. Over pints of locally brewed draught beer we plotted our surprise appearance at the Brabeck house in Carmel Valley. Lisi had arranged to keep Steve at home working in the kitchen that afternoon. We were sure that he had no inkling of the events that were about to unfold over the next thirty-six hours.

As we stole into their house, we passed the old Steinway that had belonged to our parents. That stately old piano, on which Mom, gone nearly ten years now, had filled our house so often with strains of the *Appassionata*, the *Pathetique*, and other Beethoven favorites, had found a new home in Carmel Valley. We crept quietly through the living room to the kitchen door. We stood there silently, motionless and expectant, watching Steve work at the kitchen sink preparing crabs for dinner that evening. He raised his glance from the pile of red claws in the sink, briefly looked at us, and redirected his attention to the crabs. Then he looked up again, this time more slowly, blinked at the group standing not five feet from him in the kitchen doorway, and finally, confusion yielding to astonishment, exclaimed, "What the—what the heck are you guys doing here?"

Three hours later we gathered to celebrate the fifty years of Steve's life since his surgery. Among those at Los Laureles Lodge for the festive dinner were family, friends, and colleagues. One after another, they rose to relate how their lives had been touched by Steve in ways big and small. In their remarks, as the evening continued, was an undercurrent of unspoken tribute both to the tenacity of our parents in searching for an answer for Steve, and to the courage of the surgeons and other investigators who produced the miracle that returned his life to him.

The next morning we gathered in Steve and Lisi's living room for a Mass of gratitude, celebrated by Uncle Bill. Uncle Bill had always been present in our lives. He was a seminarian when I was born, and none of us boys had known life without him. He had driven to Rochester to be with Mom and Dad on the day of Steve's first surgery. Many times, while we were growing up, he had responded to Mom's calls for help while Dad was away on one of his trips. Once he drove from the Seminary to track down Pete, who had failed to return for supper from his paper route; another time, he showed up simply to fix a broken washing machine. Now he was with us again in his eighty-second year to bless this event and to share in the family's joy. As Uncle Carl, brother to him and Mom, once said of Uncle Bill, "He's always been here for us: he has hatched us, matched us, patched us, and dispatched us."

Not long after the golden jubilee celebration, Steve began to notice a change in his physical stamina. It was subtle at first. Walking uphill, even on mild inclines, was becoming more difficult. Steve and Lisi had always been avid hikers, and the hills and meadows of Garland Park, which rise in pastoral beauty behind their house in Carmel Valley, was one of their favorite destinations. At first he thought he was simply out of shape, but he soon began to notice that even his usual gym workouts were becoming taxing. Eventually he stopped accepting invitations to go hiking with friends because it was too embarrassing to lag behind the group. "If I had a really good day I could probably do it," he said, "but my good days were becoming fewer and fewer."

He began to suffer bouts of an irregular heart rhythm, called atrial flutter. Twice he needed to have his normal heart rhythm restored by electrical cardioversion. His fatigue and shortness of breath, which he once described to me as "suffocation, like drowning," increased. Lisi was becoming worried, and began to press Steve to "do something."

Restoration

Over the years, Steve had been evaluated at the UCLA Medical Center, Stanford University Medical Center, and the Mayo Clinic, each of which has a program in adult congenital heart disease. Now he returned, seeking advice. Doctors at UCLA had wanted him to have his nonfunctional pulmonary valve replaced two years earlier. The specialists at Stanford told him that, based upon the normal echocardiographic appearance of his right ventricle, surgery was not yet necessary. Faced with conflicting advice, he trusted his intuition. His condition was spiraling downward, and he, too, knew that he needed something done. "I decided to go back to where it all began," he says. Fifty-one years after his first surgery, Steve returned to the Mayo Clinic. There, Dr. Carol Warnes, director of Mayo's Adult Congenital Heart Disease Clinic, agreed with him. A second corrective surgery was necessary. Among other planned surgical interventions, his pulmonary valve would be replaced. Steve's second operation was scheduled for the Ides of March, 2007.

The first suggestion of city that one sees when approaching Rochester from any direction is the cluster of Mayo Clinic buildings rising from the urban horizon. This city of 94,000, situated on rolling farmland just to the east of Minnesota's prairie lands, was once inhabited by nomadic Sioux, Ojibwa, and Winnebago tribes. It traces its origin to George Head, who settled on the South Fork of the Zumbro River in 1854, built himself a log cabin, and for some years operated it as Head's Tavern. He named the settlement after his home town in upstate New York. Rochester became a stagecoach stop on the road between St. Paul and Dubuque, Iowa, and its 1856 population of fifty inhabitants grew to fifteen hundred by 1858. In the early 1860s the railroad arrived, further spurring growth of the local economy and population.

In 1863, a young English physician, Dr. William Worrall Mayo, arrived in the Rochester area as a medical examiner for Union Army inductees in the Civil War. He eventually developed a frontier medical practice with his two sons, William James and Charles Horace Mayo.

In 1883, a destructive tornado leveled much of Rochester, killing thirty-seven inhabitants and leaving hundreds injured. The Doctors Mayo, assisted by the Sisters of St. Francis, a teaching order of Catholic nuns active in the area, cared for the injured survivors in a temporary infirmary quickly set up in a dance hall. Feeling acutely the inadequacy of these makeshift facilities, the elder Dr. Mayo suggested to Sister Alfred Moes, the superior of the order, that she establish a hospital in the area. "I will, if you will be its medical director," was her reply. The elder Dr. Mayo agreed, and the nuns raised $40,000 over the next four years to fund its construction. St. Marys Hospital, the original building of the complex that subsequently became the Mayo Clinic, opened its doors to receive its first patients in 1889.

The Mayo Clinic enjoys a glorious heritage and is one of the premier medical institutions in the world today. The word most closely associated with the Mayo Clinic is *excellence*—excellence in patient care, research, and teaching. Numerous innovations in medicine, surgery, physiology, epidemiology, and in the organization and delivery of health care have originated there. The Mayo Clinic was the first medical group practice in the United States. Among its more notable scientific achievements was the discovery of the hormone cortisone, for which two Mayo Clinic researchers received the Nobel Prize in Medicine and Physiology in 1950. The development of the heart-lung bypass machine occurred there. The first intensive care unit of any kind may have been the cardiac surgery ICU, which opened at St. Marys Hospital in 1957. The Mayo Clinic was at the forefront of innovations in telemedicine in the 1960s. In 1969 the first FDA-authorized total hip replacement in the United States was performed at the Clinic.

The core philosophy of the Mayo Clinic is articulated in its statement of the principle that underlies all aspects of clinical care delivered there: The needs of the patient come first. This, of course, constitutes the very definition of altruism: placing the interests and welfare of others before your own. The Mayo Clinic philosophy of patient care has remained unchanged since 1889.

* * *

Upon arriving in Rochester on the day before Steve's scheduled surgery, I checked into the Kahler Hotel, now called the Grand Kahler, and then set out for St. Marys Hospital. Dr. Kirklin had performed Steve's first surgery more than fifty-one years earlier at Rochester Methodist Hospital, but cardiac surgery is now done at St. Marys, about a mile north of the main Mayo campus. Dr. Joseph A. Dearani, a cardiothoracic surgeon and accomplished jazz musician, would operate on him there tomorrow.

March 14 was an unusually mild day in Minnesota, and warm breezes caressed me with hints of coming spring as I walked that afternoon along Second Street NW to St. Marys. Lisi met me in the hospital's main entrance lobby and brought me to Steve's room, where we waited for him to return from his pre-operative cardiac catheterization and electrophysiologic studies. When Steve finally arrived on a gurney, he smiled in greeting, and said softly, still a bit under the soft haze of sedation, "Mike, the guy who just did my cath—he was your resident for a month in Boston." Later he was discharged to return early the next morning for his surgery.

Steve and Lisi had rented an apartment across the street from St. Marys in anticipation of a few weeks' stay in Rochester. Steve had been told to expect to remain in the hospital for five to seven days after his procedure. That evening the three of us met at the apartment. We sat and talked, sipping a Cabernet that they had brought from the Monterey area. I thought that they might like to have this last evening alone, but both seemed eager for my company. Steve talked about meeting with his lawyer, financial advisor, and accountant back in California, in preparation for his second surgery. He joked that covering all the bases would give him the best chance of survival—leave one thing undone and his luck might run out.

He read aloud messages from his children, meant to be opened by him on the night before his operation. Anni, their oldest, sent photos of

her two children for him to look at while he recovered from the operation. Rosie, the youngest, sent a poem she had written for him called
"The Leaky Heart." Its final lines are,

> On the Ides of March, Dad's back under the knife
> For an operation to improve his quality of life.
> Unlike Caesar he will prevail,
> This particular surgeon is known not to fail.
> Dad refers to the operation as "cracking his chest"
> But I will use a gentler text.
> This operation will be the key
> To fixing a leaky heart that means so much to me.

Anticipating an early end to our evening, we emptied our glasses
and left the apartment to dine at Michael's Restaurant, a downtown
Rochester institution that has served steaks and seafood to locals and
visitors alike since 1951. Michael's had been a favorite of our parents
since the days of Steve's first surgery. I felt both sadness and nostalgia
as we entered the foyer of the restaurant that evening. I missed my
parents at that moment—Mom died in 1996 and Dad in 2001—
especially when Steve pointed to the table at which he thought they
usually sat. The three of us were floating on waves of anxiety, none of
us certain of the outcome of the next day's events—although this un-
certainty, of course, was left unspoken. Steve and I ordered Manhat-
tans in honor of Dad, who, when asked about it, would always attrib-
ute his long life of good health to "one Manhattan each evening, never
more, but *never* less." We sensed the presence of Mom and Dad and
toasted them. We felt them sitting with us in the booth.

Then Steve began to talk about how having been born with a cardiac defect had changed his life, or more precisely, how it had changed
him. He maintained that having a congenital disease can be, oddly, an
asset. Reflecting on how his condition has affected who he has become, he said, "It sort of puts you in a spot to look at life a bit differ-
ently, something not so permanent, and therefore something to take
advantage of while you can. It compels you to be a contributor, to play
on the court, not just to observe from the stands." He continued, "From

the standpoint of being a physician, it is invaluable. My illness has opened doors for me to understand the patients I deal with every day, and communication between us often becomes quite seamless. My tetralogy is truly a great blessing, and one I feel fortunate to have been born with.

"My response to an acquired disease would, I think, be different. I imagine that an acquired disease like cancer, for instance, would be much more difficult to accept. Your mind would constantly be dealing with 'what if' scenarios: what if this hadn't happened to me? For those of us with congenital defects, we had no choice. It's just a fact of life for us." Looking now at Lisi, he continued, "I have often tried to explain it this way: 'Hey, it's like looking at the fact that you have two hands. It's what you're born with— it's a normal part of you.' So for me it's not a defect, it's just who I am. As such, it's not something bad or tragic, but quite the opposite, because it has opened many wonderful doors of understanding for me, which has been especially useful in my chosen field. That's why I view it as a gift."

After the meal we said our good nights, and I walked back to the Grand Kahler.

Early the following morning, in the darkness of my unfamiliar hotel room, I gradually emerged from my dreams, strained into consciousness, and managed a squint at the blue quartz numbers on the clock radio, which read 6:15 am—time to be up.

A quick shower, coffee from a hallway vending machine, and out into the still, pre-dawn darkness of a Minnesota morning for an unexpectedly cold mile's walk to St. Marys Hospital. There I joined Steve and Lisi in a small, private room designated for patients awaiting surgery. They had arrived somewhat earlier. Steve had already undressed and was seated on a bench in his johnny, a blue and white hospital gown tied at the back. We made jokes about the johnny. When Steve is in the hospital, he is usually not the one wearing it. We chatted together. Steve needed conversation. We all needed it.

At 8:30 a nurse appeared pushing an empty wheelchair. It was time. Steve and Lisi were given a few moments of privacy. I touched Steve's shoulder, slipped away to an alcove down the hall, and waited. Presently another nurse came walking with Lisi alone to escort us to the family waiting area. Steve left in the wheelchair, headed in another direction.

Lisi and I were led into a large, pleasant, well lit room, amply furnished with desks, comfortable chairs, televisions, and internet access. Here, in the company of several other families, our waiting began. Waiting would be the theme of our day, waiting for anything—for the trill of the cell phone, for the hands on the clock to advance, for word from the operating room. Bathroom breaks and telephone conversations with family members eager for an update punctuated our day.

The Mayo Clinic has become quite effective in managing the needs of anxiously waiting family members. At Mayo, the patient's family is also considered to be a patient, and there is a commitment to everyone, whether family members or the patients themselves, to provide both comfort and accurate information delivered in a timely fashion.

Shortly after we arrived in the family waiting area, a kindly looking, middle-aged woman in blue scrubs appeared. Her ID badge indicated that she was an RN. "Hi, I'm Norma," she said, smiling as she approached Lisi with an outstretched hand. "I'll be your contact while Dr. Brabeck is in the operating room. After the surgery is finished, I'll bring you down to meet with Dr. Dearani so he can review for you how the surgery went and answer your questions. After that we'll all go to the cardiac surgery ICU so that you can see Dr, Brabeck." She proceeded to give us her cell phone and pager numbers. "If you need anything at all, call me. But I'll be in touch as the day goes on. No worries now."

Norma was as good as her word. At 9:00 she appeared to tell us that Steve had arrived in the operating room. At 9:30 she was back again: "The chest incision has been made." And at 10:00: "Dr. Brabeck is 'on pump.' " This meant that Steve was once again on cardiopulmonary bypass, the same technology, though considerably more sophisticated, that had kept him alive during his operation fifty-one years earlier. We also knew that Steve had been cooled to a temperature of less than 90F to minimize his metabolic requirements and protect his heart muscle during the operation. At 11:30 Norma returned to inform us that Steve had successfully come off the pump. During the nearly ninety minutes that the cardiopulmonary bypass system had been oxygenating his tissues, Dr. Dearani and his team gave Steve a new porcine pulmonary valve, harvested from a pig and then frozen to await its human recipient. Dearani then performed a cryo-ablation, a procedure in which electrical tracts of heart muscle are frozen to prevent subsequent disturbances of the heart rhythm. He and his team searched for, but did not find, the recurrent ventricular septal defect that Steve himself had previously demonstrated by echocardiography. Norma returned once again around noon to inform us that the Dr. Dearani was pleased, that all had gone well, and that the surgical team was at that moment closing Steve's chest incision.

At this point Lisi and I were still in the waiting room, anxiously awaiting our post-operation conference with Dr. Dearani. A short time later, we were brought by Norma to a consultation room near the cardiac surgery ICU. Our meeting with Dr. Dearani was brief. He has dark good looks, well maintained into the early middle years of his life. His hands are long, slender, and demonstrative. His manner that afternoon was earnest and reassuring. He informed us that from a technical standpoint the surgery had gone well. Steve's platelet count had dipped to 40,000 during the procedure (not unusual during cardio-pulmonary bypass), but there had been no excessive bleeding. Unexpectedly, a few air bubbles had been spotted in the arterial line proceeding from the bypass machine. Bubbles of air in the arterial system can be dangerous, because if they pass to the cerebral circulation they can cause a stroke. While he did not think this complication had occurred, he planned to awaken Steve early from his anesthetic sleep, just to make sure that he could move his fingers and toes.

Lisi and I were escorted to Steve's bedside in the ICU. The curtain was drawn back for us, exposing Steve's upper torso, his arms, neck, and face, which were bloated. The sight of a person in the critical care setting of a medical or surgical ICU can be disquieting for those not accustomed to it. In the post-surgical state the body is often swollen, so that the person protruding from under the sheets may little resemble the one you said good-by to mere hours ago. Typically there are several tubes that seem to enter or exit every body orifice, in addition to various intravenous and arterial lines. Add to this the visual impact of multiple screens monitoring vital signs, heart rhythm, and respiratory parameters, and all their associated beeps and alarms, and the picture can become quickly confusing, and even frightening.

Steve's nurse temporarily stopped the intravenous sedative. He awakened briefly and felt Lisi's warm breath on his cheek. On command he pressed his fingers into her hand, first on the right and then the left. He wiggled the toes of both feet. The sedative was restarted.

Then we both relaxed. Steve had awakened, recognized Lisi, and moved everything appropriately. With Steve asleep again, his nurse directed Lisi's attention to a small table at the foot of the bed, where Steve's old medical record from 1955 was folded into a half-size manila envelope. "Take a look in there," he said. "You'll be surprised."

Lisi reached for the envelope and extracted its contents. She examined the few sheets of yellowed paper containing type- and handwritten clinical notes more than a half-century old, and found a Christmas card stapled to them. As she read, she began to cry quietly. She handed me the card, a season's greeting written in my mother's hand, dated December 15, 1956, just over a year after Steve's initial operation. It read:

> *Dear Dr. Kirklin,*
>
> *It is probably superfluous to tell you that Stevie is in 'A No. 1' shape this winter.*
>
> *He is leading a new life, and still now and then refers to the fact that Dr. Kirklin's 'operation' makes all this possible for him.*
>
> *Again, may we express our gratitude to you? We can never forget.*
>
> *Sincerely,*
> *(signed) George and Marie Brabeck*

Two days later I left Rochester and headed back home to New York City. Steve was discharged from St. Marys after five days. He and Lisi spent several additional days in Rochester in their rented apartment, making follow-up surveillance visits at the Clinic.

On the morning of their final day in Rochester, while preparing to leave their apartment for the last time, Steve suddenly felt drawn to visit the chapel in St. Marys Hospital. "I don't know why I needed to go there," he recalls. "It was just something I felt I had to do." Lisi accompanied him. They crossed the street and entered the hospital. St. Marys Hospital Chapel is situated within the hospital complex and was designed as a basilica in elegant Italian Renaissance style. With the capacity to seat four hundred worshipers, it is impressively large for a hospital chapel.

Settling in one of the rear pews, Steve and Lisi sat in silence, Steve alone in his thoughts. "As I sat there, Mom spoke to me," he later told me. I asked Steve if he saw her, and he answered no, he did not. But he continued, "Mom told me, in her voice 'I can go now, it's okay.' " Clearly feeling the intense intimacy of the encounter, he did not wish to describe it further.

Steve and Lisi flew back to California on March 31. By mid-April, Steve was back in his office seeing patients again (and yes, taking night call!).

The Question

The exertions of many surgeons, cardiologists, and other investigators, who for years had been laboring toward the goal of operating inside the heart, formed the foundation for the efforts of Kirklin and Lillehei. But only these two surgeons were actually operating on patients at the dawn of open heart surgery. It was they who developed the early technology for cardiopulmonary bypass: first, controlled cross-circulation and later, the Mayo-Gibbon heart-lung bypass machine and the DeWall-Lillehei oxygenator. And it was on their patients, most of them Minnesota residents, that the technology was refined so that it could be exported to other medical centers. In the mid-1950s, following the published accounts of these early surgeries, cardiopulmonary bypass technology exploded into the world beyond Minnesota. The first truly commercial heart-lung machine was the Mayo-Gibbon device, which was the most widely used heart-lung machine during the 1950s and early 1960s.

With the rising numbers of open heart procedures done in the United States and elsewhere—in 2004, 646,000 open heart procedures were done in the US alone—the risk of dying in the intra- or postoperative period has steadily declined. In 1955, the operative mortality associated with curative surgical repair of Tetralogy of Fallot was fifty percent. By 1960, that number had plummeted to fifteen percent. In 1980, the risk of dying during or after open heart surgery was under two percent, and in some medical centers approached zero. Anesthetic and surgical techniques continue to be refined. Today, the mortality risk from cardiac surgery depends primarily on patient's non-cardiac conditions and on the health of the heart muscle itself.

With Steve's surgery successfully completed, I returned to my own practice at Bellevue. Once again engaged in my busy world of patients, residents, and medical students, I began to muse about why

Steve had gotten more than fifty-one years of good, active life out of his original surgery. I had never really thought about this before.

Most children who have had a Tetralogy of Fallot repaired will eventually need a second heart operation. That is because pressure increases over time in the right ventricle, the consequence of a chronically malfunctioning pulmonary valve, which controls the flow of blood to the lungs. As pressure builds, the right ventricle dilates and becomes overloaded, and the patient begins to retain fluid in tissues outside of the vascular system. This is manifest as swollen legs, liver congestion, or an abdomen protuberant with extra fluid.

But Steve's right ventricle had never failed, and I wondered why. Steve has a theory about this. His repair had been done in the early days of open heart surgery, before surgeons realized that the heart muscle, the myocardium, could be protected from injury during bypass procedures. Today, myocardial protection is accomplished by chilling the patient to temperatures of 90 degrees Fahrenheit or less during surgery. This slows down tissue metabolism, rendering the heart and other vital tissues less susceptible to injury during anesthesia and bypass, when periods of fluctuating blood pressure or oxygen tension may occur. But in the 1950s these techniques had yet to be developed. Steve thinks that because he did not have the benefit of myocardial protection, scarring occurred in his heart muscle. Called myocardial fibrosis, this may have prevented his right ventricle from dilating over the ensuing years and eventually failing. What finally got Steve into trouble was not right ventricular failure, but progressively decreasing cardiac output. Paradoxically, that same scarring which probably protected his right ventricle, also limited its ability to receive blood from the venous system. His heart was just not receiving enough blood to pump forward to the lungs and the rest of the body. Once again, as in his childhood, Steve's heart was unable to keep apace with the physiologic demands of his body.

Waiting near the bank of elevators on the seventeenth floor of Bellevue late one afternoon, I encountered Bill Slater, a clinical cardiologist on the faculty of New York University School of Medicine who is based at the hospital. Broad shouldered and of medium stature, Bill has a natural physical grace about him. His easygoing smile belies a keen intellect and unmatched clinical astuteness. For more than a generation he has been revered and loved by patients and students of medicine at every level.

I was still puzzled by the longevity of Steve's original surgical correction, and explained Steve's idea to him. Bill listened carefully and considered the hypothesis. A grin spread over his face, which faded into a soft smile as he lowered his gaze to the polished tiled floor, or perhaps to the toes of his shoes. "You may be right," he reflected with a shrug, "but I think God was on his side."

"Come on, Bill. You're a cardiologist!"

"I know," he repeated, pushing the down button. "But God was on his side."

An Open Heart

On the evening of April 25, little more than a month after his second surgery, I received a telephone call from Steve. I sensed immediately he had *animo*, good energy. "Mike, he said, "I had a banner day today, and I want to tell you about it. This morning I was taking my walk with Kobe [the family dog], and instead of heading left down Via Las Encinas [a country road near his house], we took a right, which heads us directly up the hill to the take-off of the Mesa trail in Garland Park. The Mesa trail is not a particularly strenuous hike, but it is about a three-mile round trip, and the first one and a half miles is progressively uphill, sometimes at a rather steep grade. This has always been one of my favorite hikes, always a relaxer for me. It takes you up to an elevation of about 700 feet and opens to a beautiful, expansive meadow surrounded by a live oak forest. The first flank of the Santa Lucia mountains, which are cloaked in a vibrant oak forest, rises abruptly from the opposite side of the meadow. It's quiet up there and serene, and the views of the valley are beautiful. It also is a hike I haven't been able to do for more than half a year, as it became just too much of a struggle for me. Today I made it with almost no problem. It was my first time climbing the trail in many months, and, Mike, I didn't really have to pace myself that much. Amazing, considering that my body struggled only three weeks ago with any rise over five feet.

"Anyhow, the day was beautiful! It was a day to marvel and give thanks for this body of mine and for how I was born. I was given two gifts at birth: my family and my Tetralogy. My defective heart and its repair now make me appreciate so much the special moments we all are handed in any given day. To me it's a bonus: I don't have to worry about taking things for granted. I was close to losing it all, and actually had come to some acceptance of that, if that was what was to be. But to experience what I did today is miraculous, like a rebirth. I feel like a bird born without wings that was given a set, then slowly lost them, and now has had them returned again. It's hard to communicate how wonderful it feels, and the deep sense of appreciation for everything in my life that it spawns."

Later, I wished I had asked Steve to write down everything that he had experienced that day. But a few days afterward I received the following e-mail from him.

"The day was all about sights, sounds, smells, and feelings. Horizon to horizon the sky was cloudless, a deep blue. The 'ghost riders' were out—silver wave on green wave of tall meadow grasses, rhythmic, blown by the wind, rippling and alternating, one long line after another, long lines of horse-mounted Indians riding through the meadows before the wind. Every spring I love that image, and I really do feel that someone is there.

"Deep purple fields of small bush lupines; the more subtle, delicate blue of the anemones; the intense spring green of the new shoot growth of the live oaks, and the green, flowing cloak of trees that covers them. There's a wisp of a shadow overhead—a red tail hawk gliding by, watching for prey in the grass below.

"The sounds of the mesa are subtle, but so obvious to one who will listen. Shuffling dust and gravel of the trail; the dry whoosh of long stem grass against your pants; the buzzing of bees in the flowering ceonanthus (I wonder where their hive was); the sharp chirp of the lone red tail hawk overhead; the muffled fluttering of the kite's wings as it hovers mid-air above the grasses, intent on any field mouse that might scurry below; and the rise and the fall of the blowing wind, almost rhythmic, like a seashore. These are mesa sounds, and it's been so long since I've heard them.

"The smells are the scents of fresh spring: the grass and trees dry in the meadow, the soft, musty moss of the forest."

Reading on, I slowed a bit, aware of a slight struggle in my throat and of moisture forming in my eyes. I continued as a single tear traced a downward path on my cheek.

"Mike, I didn't miss a thing yesterday. It was probably the most mindful I've ever been. I just appreciated everything around me so much. My senses were not overloaded, just aware and receptive.

Again, it comes from the gift I've been given—I wouldn't trade it for the world. Our bodies are truly wonders, and the environment in which we exist is only what we make of it, which means it can be miraculous any time we let it be."

Today, at age 59, Steve Brabeck is probably the longest-living survivor of surgical correction of Tetralogy of Fallot. Some may say that's a result of near-perfect timing: he was born in St. Paul, just as open-heart surgery was dawning at the Mayo Clinic and at nearby University of Minnesota. But there's another way to look at it. Open heart surgery attained viability at that time in history because of the difficult, unrelenting, brilliant work of surgeons like John Gibbon, John W. Kirklin, and C. Walton Lillehei. Steve entered the early trials of this surgery because a tight-knit community of concerned friends and relatives were constantly alert to medical advances that might help him. My parents managed Steve's illness as they managed all family matters, with wisdom and grace and love. And growing up in their care enabled all their sons, especially Steve, to understand that his Tetralogy, that any challenge, could be a source of strength, a spur to live life fully, generously, with heart, open to the possibility of miracles. Finally, I think that Bill Slater got it right. God *was* on Steve's side.

I wish to acknowledge the editorial assistance of Ms. Kitty Barnes in the preparation of this manuscript, and express my profound gratitude for her contributions.

www.ingramcontent.com/pod-product-compliance
Lightning Source LLC
Chambersburg PA
CBHW031327290526
45784CB00014B/2412